Mindful Self-Care Approaches

Susan Rogers

HSC Training Link

DEDICATION

This book is dedicated to all those looking for a work-life balance, for those wanting a more relaxed way of life, for those wanting to deal with stress in an effective way and for the curious.

CONTENTS

ACKNOWLEDGMENTS

Self-Care Forum: https://www.selfcareforum.org/
Anna Freud Centre: https://www.annafreud.org/on-my-mind/self-care/
National Institute of Mental Health: https://www.nimh.nih.gov/health/topics/caring-for-your-mental-health
MIND: https://www.mind.org.uk/information-support/types-of-mental-health-problems/mental-health-problems-introduction/self-care/

1 MINDFUL SELF-CARE APPROACHES

Looking after yourself from a mindfulness approach involves cultivating a deeper awareness of your thoughts, emotions and bodily sensations in the present moment without judgment.

Mindfulness is a practice rooted in ancient Buddhist traditions but has gained popularity in recent years as a way to reduce stress, improve well-being and enhance overall mental and emotional health.

Here are some key principles and practices associated with looking after yourself from a mindfulness perspective:

- **Present Moment Awareness:**
  - Mindfulness encourages you to pay full attention to the present moment.
  - Often, we're lost in thoughts about the past or future, which can lead to stress and anxiety.
  - By focusing on the "here and now," you can better manage your thoughts and reactions.

- **Non-Judgmental Observation:**
  - Mindfulness involves observing your thoughts, feelings and sensations without judgment.
  - Instead of labelling experiences as good or bad, try to accept them as they are.
  - This non-judgmental attitude helps reduce self-criticism and self-blame.

- **Breath Awareness:**
  - One of the most common mindfulness practices is mindful breathing.
  - Paying attention to your breath as it goes in and out can anchor you in the present moment, calm your mind and regulate your emotions.

- **Body Scan:**
  - A body scan involves systematically directing your attention to different parts of your body, noticing any sensations, tension or discomfort.
  - This practice can help you become more aware of physical sensations and release bodily tension.

- **Mindful Eating:**
  - Eating mindfully involves savouring each bite, paying attention to the taste, texture and smell of your food.
  - This practice can help prevent overeating and promote a healthier relationship with food.

- **Mindful Walking:**
  - When you walk mindfully, you pay close attention to the sensation of each step, your surroundings and the rhythm of your walking.
  - It's a great way to connect with nature and reduce

stress.

- **Meditation:**

  - Mindfulness meditation is a formal practice that involves sitting in a quiet place and focusing on your breath, bodily sensations or a specific object.

  - Meditation helps train your mind to stay present and cultivate mindfulness.

- **Self-Compassion:**

  - Mindfulness encourages self-compassion, which involves treating yourself with the same kindness and understanding that you would offer to a friend.

  - It's about being gentle with yourself, especially in challenging moments.

- **Stress Reduction:**

  - By practising mindfulness regularly, you can reduce the impact of stress on your life.

  - Mindfulness helps you become more resilient and better able to cope with difficult situations.

- **Improved Emotional Regulation:**

  - Mindfulness can help you better understand and regulate your emotions.

  - By observing your feelings without judgment, you can respond to them in healthier ways.

- **Enhanced Well-Being:**

  - Over time, mindfulness can lead to increased overall well-being, greater happiness and a deeper sense of inner peace.

Remember that mindfulness is a skill that takes time to develop. Consistent practice is key to experiencing its benefits.

You can start with short sessions and gradually increase the duration as you become more comfortable with the practice.

There are also many resources available, including books, apps and guided meditation sessions, to support your mindfulness journey.

2 PRESENT MOMENT AWARENESS

Present Moment Awareness, often simply referred to as "being present" or "living in the moment," is a core concept in mindfulness and a fundamental aspect of mindfulness practice.

It involves focusing your attention on the here and now, fully immersing yourself in your current experience and letting go of distractions, worries or preoccupations about the past or future.

Here are some key aspects and benefits of present moment awareness:

- **Non-Judgmental Observation:**
  - When you practice present moment awareness, you observe your thoughts, emotions and sensations without judgment.
  - Instead of labelling them as good or bad, you simply notice them as they arise.
  - This non-judgmental attitude can help reduce self-criticism and promote self-acceptance.

- **Reduced Stress and Anxiety:**
  - Many of our stressors and anxieties stem from ruminating on the past or worrying about the future.
  - By grounding yourself in the present moment, you can break free from these patterns of thought and experience a sense of calm and relaxation.

- **Improved Concentration:**
  - When you give your full attention to the task at hand, your concentration and focus naturally improve.
  - This can enhance your productivity and the quality of your work or activities.

- **Enhanced Relationships:**
  - Being fully present when interacting with others can lead to better communication and deeper connections.
  - It shows that you value the person you're with and that you're actively listening and engaged in the conversation.

- **Appreciation and Gratitude:**
  - Present moment awareness can help you appreciate the simple joys and beauty in everyday life.
  - It encourages a sense of gratitude for the present moment, even during challenging times.

- **Mindful Decision-Making:**
  - When you make decisions with full awareness of the present moment, you're less likely to react impulsively or be swayed by automatic, habitual patterns of thinking.
  - This can lead to wiser and more intentional choices.

- **Enhanced Physical Sensations:**
  - Being present allows you to fully experience physical sensations.
  - Whether it's savouring the taste of your food, feeling the warmth of the sun on your skin or enjoying the sensation of a hug, you can derive greater pleasure from your sensory experiences.

- **Mindful Stress Management:**
  - In stressful situations, practising present moment awareness can help you respond rather than react.
  - You can assess the situation more objectively and choose how to respond in a way that aligns with your values and goals.

- **Cultivation of Mindfulness:**
  - Present moment awareness is a foundational practice in cultivating overall mindfulness.
  - When you learn to stay present, it becomes easier to integrate mindfulness into other aspects of your life.

To cultivate present moment awareness in your daily life, you can start with simple practices such as mindful breathing, where you focus your attention on your breath as it goes in and out.

Additionally, you can bring mindfulness to routine activities like eating, walking or even washing dishes by fully engaging your senses and thoughts in those moments.

Remember that present moment awareness is a skill that requires regular practice. It's common for the mind to wander, but each time you notice it has wandered, gently bring your attention back to the present moment without self-criticism.

Over time, you'll find it easier to stay present and reap the benefits of this practice.

3 NON-JUDGEMENTAL OBSERVATION

Non-judgmental observation, a core principle of mindfulness, involves observing your thoughts, emotions and sensory experiences without evaluating, criticising or attaching value judgments to them.

Instead of labelling these experiences as good or bad, right or wrong, you aim to simply notice them as they arise, accepting them as part of your present reality.

Here's more information on non-judgmental observation:

- **Radical Acceptance:**
  - Non-judgmental observation often goes hand in hand with the concept of radical acceptance.
  - This means fully acknowledging and accepting your present experience, no matter how uncomfortable or challenging it may be.
  - By doing so, you allow yourself to be with what is, rather than resisting or fighting against it.

- **Reduced Self-Criticism:**
  - Many people have a tendency to be overly critical of themselves.

- When you practice non-judgmental observation, you create a space where self-criticism can decrease.
- Instead of berating yourself for feeling a certain way or having particular thoughts, you simply observe them with curiosity and compassion.

- **Increased Self-Awareness:**
  - Non-judgmental observation enhances your self-awareness by providing a clearer view of your internal landscape.
  - You become more attuned to your thoughts, emotions and bodily sensations, which can help you understand yourself better and make conscious choices.

- **Emotional Regulation:**
  - Observing your emotions without judgment can be particularly helpful for emotional regulation.
  - When you allow emotions to be present without resisting or reacting impulsively, they often naturally subside.
  - This can prevent emotional outbursts or impulsive behaviours.

- **Enhanced Objectivity:**
  - Non-judgmental observation promotes objectivity.
  - By not immediately categorising experiences as positive or negative, you can approach situations with a more balanced and open perspective.
  - This can lead to more effective problem-solving and decision-making.

- **Mindful Communication:**
  - In relationships, non-judgmental observation can

improve communication.

- When you listen without judgment to what others are saying, you create a safe space for open dialogue and understanding.

- This can foster deeper connections with others.

- **Stress Reduction:**

  - The practice of non-judgmental observation can be particularly effective in reducing stress.

  - When you let go of the need to judge or control your experiences, you can find greater peace and calm in the midst of life's challenges.

- **Freedom from Automatic Reactions:**

  - By observing your thoughts and emotions without judgment, you gain greater freedom from automatic reactions.

  - Instead of being driven by habitual responses, you can choose how to respond more intentionally to situations.

- **Mindful Problem-Solving:**

  - When you encounter problems or difficulties, non-judgmental observation can help you approach them with a clear and open mind.

  - This can lead to more creative and effective solutions.

- **Enhanced Compassion:**

  - Non-judgmental observation of your own experiences can extend to greater compassion for yourself and others.

  - When you realise that everyone experiences thoughts

and emotions without judgment, it becomes easier to relate to others with empathy and kindness.

To practice non-judgmental observation, start by simply noticing your thoughts, emotions and sensations as they arise.

When you catch yourself making judgments, gently redirect your attention to the act of observing.

Over time, this practice can become a valuable tool for enhancing your mindfulness, self-awareness and overall well-being.

4 BREATH AWARENESS

Breath awareness is a foundational mindfulness practice that involves focusing your attention on the breath, observing it as it moves in and out of your body.

It is a simple yet powerful technique that can have profound effects on your mental, emotional and physical well-being.

Here's more information about breath awareness:

- **Anchor to the Present Moment:**
  - Your breath is always with you in the present moment.
  - By directing your attention to your breath, you bring your awareness to the here and now, helping you let go of distractions, worries and anxieties about the past or future.

- **Calm and Relaxation:**
  - Focusing on your breath can induce a sense of calm and relaxation.
  - Deep, mindful breathing activates the body's parasympathetic nervous system, which counteracts the "fight-or-flight" stress response, promoting

relaxation and reducing stress.

- **Awareness of the Body:**
  - Breath awareness often begins with noticing the physical sensations associated with breathing.
  - You might feel the rise and fall of your chest or the expansion and contraction of your abdomen.
  - This enhances your body awareness.

- **Observing Thoughts and Emotions:**
  - As you practice breath awareness, you may notice that your mind frequently wanders, getting caught up in thoughts, worries or distractions.
  - This is normal.
  - The practice encourages you to gently acknowledge these mental wanderings and return your focus to your breath without self-criticism.

- **Enhanced Concentration:**
  - Regular practice of breath awareness can improve your concentration and focus.
  - This enhanced concentration can spill over into other aspects of your life, such as work or study.

- **Emotional Regulation:**
  - Breath awareness is a valuable tool for managing emotions.
  - When you observe your breath, you can become more aware of emotional responses as they arise.
  - This awareness allows you to respond to emotions more skilfully rather than reacting impulsively.

- **Stress Reduction:**
    - Mindful breathing can be an effective stress reduction technique.
    - It can help you become more resilient in the face of stressors, allowing you to respond to challenging situations with greater equanimity.

- **Improved Sleep:**
    - Practising breath awareness before bedtime can help calm racing thoughts and promote better sleep.
    - A relaxed mind and body are more conducive to restful sleep.

- **Mind-Body Connection:**
    - Breath awareness deepens your connection to your body.
    - It can help you become more attuned to physical sensations, which can be useful for managing chronic pain or discomfort.

- **Enhanced Mindfulness Practice:**
    - Breath awareness is often used as a foundational practice to develop overall mindfulness.
    - As you become more adept at focusing on your breath, you can extend this mindfulness to other aspects of your life, such as eating, walking or working.

To practice breath awareness:

- Find a quiet and comfortable place to sit or lie down.

- Close your eyes if you're comfortable doing so.

- Bring your attention to your breath. Notice the sensation of the breath as it enters and leaves your nostrils or the rise and fall of your chest or abdomen.

- If your mind wanders (which it likely will), gently bring your focus back to your breath without judgment.

- Continue this practice for a predetermined amount of time, such as 5 to 10 minutes to start, gradually increasing the duration as you become more comfortable with the practice.

Remember that breath awareness is a skill that develops with consistent practice.

Over time, you may notice the positive effects it has on your overall well-being and mindfulness.

5 BODY SCAN AWARENESS

The body scan is a mindfulness meditation practice that involves systematically directing your attention to different parts of your body, typically from head to toe or vice versa.

The aim is to become more aware of bodily sensations, tensions and areas of relaxation without judgment.

Here's more information about the body scan practice:

- **Deepening Mindfulness:**

  - The body scan is an effective way to deepen your mindfulness practice.

  - It enhances your ability to observe sensations, thoughts and emotions as they arise in the body, helping you develop a more profound sense of self-awareness.

- **Stress Reduction:**

  - The body scan can be particularly helpful for reducing stress and promoting relaxation.

  - It allows you to become aware of areas of tension in the body and consciously release them, leading to a greater sense of calm and physical relaxation.

- **Physical Awareness:**
  - Through the body scan, you can become more attuned to physical sensations and any discomfort or pain you might be experiencing.
  - This heightened awareness can be valuable for managing chronic pain or physical discomfort.

- **Emotional Regulation:**
  - As you scan your body, you may notice that certain areas are associated with emotional tension or discomfort.
  - This connection between physical sensations and emotions can be insightful and help you regulate your emotional responses more effectively.

- **Non-Judgmental Observation:**
  - Similar to other mindfulness practices, the body scan encourages non-judgmental observation.
  - Rather than labelling sensations as good or bad, you aim to observe them without evaluation, fostering self-compassion and acceptance.

- **Increased Body Connection:**
  - The body scan strengthens the mind-body connection.
  - It can help you recognise how stress or emotions manifest physically in your body and give you tools to address these manifestations in a healthy way.

- **Improved Sleep:**
  - Engaging in a body scan before bedtime can help calm the mind and body, making it easier to fall asleep and experience more restful sleep.

- **Reduced Muscle Tension:**

  - By systematically scanning for areas of tension and consciously releasing them, you can reduce physical discomfort caused by muscle tension and tightness.

- **Enhanced Self-Care:**

  - Practising the body scan is a form of self-care.

  - It provides you with an opportunity to check in with yourself, notice any areas of discomfort or stress and take steps to address them, promoting overall well-being.

To practice the body scan:

- Find a quiet and comfortable place to lie down on your back. You can use a yoga mat, a blanket or a comfortable surface.

- Close your eyes and take a few deep breaths to relax.

- Begin the scan at the top of your head or the tips of your toes, depending on your preference. Slowly and systematically move your attention through each part of your body.

- As you focus on each area, pay attention to any sensations you notice, such as warmth, tension, tingling or relaxation. There's no need to change anything; simply observe.

- If you encounter areas of tension, try to relax them as best you can by consciously releasing any held tension and breathing into that area.

- Continue scanning your body until you reach the toes or head, depending on where you began.

- Take a few moments to notice your body as a whole, your breath and your overall state of relaxation.

- When you're ready, gently open your eyes and bring your awareness back to the present moment.

The body scan can be adapted to different lengths, ranging from a short 5-minute practice to a more extended 20-30 minute session.

Consistent practice can deepen your mindfulness skills and help you become more in tune with your body and emotions.

6 MINDFUL EATING AWARENESS

Mindful eating is a practice that encourages you to pay full attention to the experience of eating, bringing a heightened awareness to the flavours, textures, smells and overall enjoyment of your food.

It involves being fully present during meals, savouring each bite and making conscious choices about what and how you eat.

Here's more information about mindful eating:

- **Slower Eating:**
    - Mindful eating often involves slowing down your eating pace.
    - By taking your time with each bite, you give your body a chance to signal when it's full, which can help prevent overeating and promote better digestion.

- **Increased Enjoyment:**
    - When you eat mindfully, you can derive greater pleasure from your meals.
    - By fully savouring the tastes and textures of your food, you can experience a deeper sense of satisfaction.

- **Improved Digestion:**
  - Eating slowly and mindfully can aid in digestion.
  - Chewing your food thoroughly and paying attention to the process of eating can help your body break down food more effectively.

- **Reduced Emotional Eating:**
  - Mindful eating can help you become more aware of emotional eating patterns, such as eating when stressed, bored or anxious.
  - This awareness allows you to make healthier choices and address emotional triggers more effectively.

- **Enhanced Awareness of Hunger and Fullness:**
  - Mindful eating helps you become attuned to your body's hunger and fullness cues.
  - This can prevent overeating or undereating and promote a healthier relationship with food.

- **Conscious Food Choices:**
  - Mindful eating encourages you to make conscious choices about what you eat.
  - You may become more selective about the foods you consume, choosing those that nourish your body and align with your values.

- **Mindful Food Preparation:**
  - The practice of mindful eating can extend to the preparation of meals.
  - Being fully present while cooking or preparing food can enhance the overall eating experience.

- **Mindful Snacking:**
  - It's not just about meals; mindful eating can be applied to snacking as well.
  - Instead of mindlessly munching on snacks, you can bring awareness to the flavours and sensations of each bite.

- **Gratitude and Appreciation:**
  - Mindful eating encourages a sense of gratitude for the food you have and the effort that went into producing it.
  - It promotes a deeper connection to the sources of your food and the Earth.

- **Reduced Stress and Anxiety:**
  - Eating mindfully can reduce stress and anxiety related to food choices.
  - By making conscious decisions and savouring your meals, you can avoid guilt or anxiety associated with impulsive or unhealthy eating habits.

- **Weight Management:**
  - Some studies suggest that practising mindful eating may be helpful for weight management because it can lead to a more balanced approach to food, reducing the likelihood of overindulgence or restrictive dieting.

To practice mindful eating:

- **Create a Calm Environment**: Find a quiet, comfortable place to eat without distractions like the TV or computer.

- **Observe Your Food**: Take a moment to look at your food, appreciating its colours, textures and presentation.

- **Engage Your Senses**: As you eat, pay attention to the taste, smell and texture of each bite. Notice the flavours and how they change as you chew.

- **Chew Thoroughly**: Chew your food slowly and thoroughly. This aids digestion and allows you to savoir each bite.

- **Put Down Utensils**: Between bites, put down your utensils or food and take a breath. This helps you avoid rushing through your meal.

- **Listen to Your Body**: Pay attention to hunger and fullness cues. Eat until you're satisfied, not overly full.

- **Practice Gratitude**: Take a moment to express gratitude for the food you're eating and the nourishment it provides.

Mindful eating is a practice that can be integrated into your daily life to promote a healthier relationship with food, reduce overeating and enhance the overall enjoyment of meals.

It's about being present with your food and making conscious choices that align with your well-being.

7 MINDFUL WALKING AWARENESS

Mindful walking, also known as walking meditation, is a mindfulness practice that involves walking slowly and deliberately while paying close attention to each step and the sensations associated with the act of walking.

It's a way to bring mindfulness into motion and can be a valuable practice for promoting relaxation, reducing stress and deepening your connection to the present moment.

Here's more information about mindful walking:

- **Slowing Down:**
    - Mindful walking is typically done at a slower pace than regular walking.
    - The intention is not to reach a destination quickly but to savoir each step and the experience of walking itself.

- **Connection to Nature:**
    - Mindful walking is often practices in natural settings like parks, gardens or along a scenic trail.
    - Being in nature can enhance the practice by allowing

you to connect with the environment and appreciate the beauty around you.

- **Body Awareness:**
  - As you walk mindfully, you bring your attention to the physical sensations of walking.
  - This includes feeling the ground beneath your feet, the movement of your legs, the sway of your arms and the rhythm of your breath.

- **Breath Awareness:**
  - Mindful walking often involves coordinating your breath with your steps.
  - You might take a breath with each step, syncing your inhalation and exhalation with your walking rhythm.

- **Mindful Observing:**
  - In addition to focusing on your body and breath, you can also practice mindful observing.
  - This means paying attention to the sights, sounds and smells around you without attachment or judgment.

- **Stress Reduction:**
  - Mindful walking can be a powerful tool for reducing stress and promoting relaxation.
  - It helps you break away from the fast-paced, multitasking mindset and guides you to a calmer and more centred state.

- **Improved Concentration:**
  - Just like other mindfulness practices, mindful walking enhances your concentration and focus.
  - It encourages you to bring your attention back to the present moment whenever your mind starts to

wander.

- **Enhanced Awareness:**
  - Mindful walking can heighten your overall awareness.
  - You may notice subtleties in your surroundings that you usually overlook, as well as a greater awareness of your own physical sensations and emotions.

- **Emotional Regulation:**
  - Practising mindfulness while walking can help you become more aware of your emotions and how they manifest in your body.
  - This can be particularly helpful for managing stress or difficult emotions.

- **Entering and Grounding:**
  - Mindful walking can serve as a grounding practice. It connects you to the earth and can help you feel more centred and balanced.

To practice mindful walking:

- Find a quiet and safe place to walk. This can be indoors or outdoors, but it should be free from distractions and obstacles.

- Begin by standing still for a moment and taking a few deep breaths to centre yourself.

- Start walking slowly and deliberately, paying close attention to each step. You can walk in a straight line or in a small, designated area.

- Focus on the physical sensations of walking—the lifting of your foot, the swinging of your leg, the contact with the ground and so on.

- Coordinate your breath with your steps if it feels natural to you, taking a breath with each step.

- If your mind starts to wander or you become distracted, gently bring your attention back to the act of walking and your breath.

- As you walk, be mindful of your surroundings, observing the sights, sounds and smells without judgment.

- Continue walking mindfully for a predetermined amount of time, such as 10-15 minutes or longer if you prefer.

Mindful walking is a practice that can be adapted to your preferences and needs.

It's a simple yet profound way to integrate mindfulness into your daily life and experience the benefits of being fully present in each moment.

8 MEDITATION AWARENESS

Meditation is a diverse and ancient practice that encompasses a wide range of techniques and traditions, all aimed at cultivating mindfulness, concentration, relaxation and a heightened state of awareness.

Here's more information about meditation:

- **Diverse Practices:**
  - Meditation is not a one-size-fits-all practice.
  - There are numerous meditation techniques, including mindfulness meditation, loving-kindness meditation, transcendental meditation, Zen meditation, Vipassana and many others.
  - Each technique has its own unique focus and approach.

- **Mindfulness Meditation:**
  - One of the most widely practised forms of meditation is mindfulness meditation.
  - It involves paying non-judgmental attention to your thoughts, emotions and bodily sensations as they arise in the present moment.

- Mindfulness meditation is often used for stress reduction, emotional regulation and improving overall well-being.

- **Concentration Meditation:**

  - Concentration meditation techniques involve focusing your attention on a single point of focus, such as your breath, a mantra, a candle flame or a specific image.

  - The aim is to train the mind to become more concentrated and less distracted.

- **Transcendental Meditation:**

  - Transcendental Meditation (TM) is a specific meditation technique that involves silently repeating a mantra.

  - TM practitioners believe that this technique can lead to a transcendent state of consciousness and deep relaxation.

1. **Loving-Kindness Meditation:**

   - Also known as Metta meditation, this practice involves generating feelings of love, compassion and goodwill towards oneself and others.

   - It's used to cultivate feelings of kindness and empathy.

- **Vipassana Meditation:**

  - Vipassana is an ancient form of meditation that involves observing the sensations in the body to gain insight into the impermanent nature of reality.

  - It's often taught in intensive retreat settings.

- **Zen Meditation:**

  - Zen meditation or Zazen, is a form of seated

meditation that emphasises simply sitting and observing the mind without attachment or aversion to thoughts.

- ◦ It's commonly associated with Zen Buddhism.

- **Health Benefits:**

  - ◦ Meditation has been extensively studied and has been found to offer a wide range of health benefits.

  - ◦ These include reduced stress, improved emotional well-being, better concentration, lowered blood pressure, improved sleep and enhanced immune function.

- **Spiritual and Philosophical Roots:**

  - ◦ Meditation has deep roots in various spiritual and philosophical traditions, including Buddhism, Hinduism, Taoism and others.

  - ◦ It's often used as a tool for spiritual growth, self-discovery and connecting with a higher consciousness or inner wisdom.

- **Scientific Research:**

  - ◦ Over the past few decades, there has been a growing interest in studying the effects of meditation from a scientific perspective.

  - ◦ Research has shown that regular meditation can lead to structural and functional changes in the brain, including increased gray matter density in areas associated with memory, learning and self-awareness.

- **Mindfulness-Based Interventions:**

  - ◦ Meditation, particularly mindfulness meditation, is used in various therapeutic and clinical settings as part of mindfulness-based interventions (MBIs).

- These interventions are designed to help individuals manage conditions like anxiety, depression, chronic pain and addiction.

- **Accessible and Flexible:**

  - One of the appealing aspects of meditation is its accessibility.

  - It can be practised almost anywhere and doesn't require special equipment.

  - You can tailor your meditation practice to fit your needs and schedule, whether you have just a few minutes or an hour to spare.

- **Regular Practice:**

  - Like any skill, meditation benefits from regular practice.

  - Consistency is key to experiencing the full range of benefits and many people find it helpful to establish a daily meditation routine.

Whether you're interested in meditation for stress reduction, personal growth, spiritual exploration or general well-being, there's likely a meditation technique that suits your preferences and goals.

It's a practice that can be deeply transformative and can lead to a greater sense of inner peace and self-awareness.

9 SELF COMPASSION AWARENESS

Self-compassion is the practice of treating oneself with the same kindness, care and understanding that one would offer to a good friend in times of suffering, failure or difficulty.

It involves being gentle with oneself and embracing one's own imperfections and humanity.

Here's more information about self-compassion:

- **Components of Self-Compassion:**
  - Self-compassion consists of three main components, as outlined by Dr. Kristin Neff, a leading researcher in the field:
    1. **Self-kindness:** Being warm and understanding toward oneself rather than self-critical or judgmental.
    2. **Common humanity:** Recognising that suffering, mistakes and challenges are a natural part of the human experience and that you're not alone in experiencing them.
    3. **Mindfulness:** Holding one's painful thoughts and feelings in balanced awareness, neither suppressing them nor exaggerating their

significance.

- **Benefits of Self-Compassion:**
  - Practising self-compassion has been linked to a range of psychological, emotional and physical benefits, including reduced levels of anxiety and depression, increased resilience, improved well-being, greater life satisfaction and better relationships with others.

- **Contrasting Self-Compassion with Self-Esteem:**
  - Self-compassion is different from self-esteem. While self-esteem is often based on judgments of self-worth and comparisons with others, self-compassion is about being kind and understanding toward yourself regardless of your perceived worth or achievements.
  - Self-compassion doesn't depend on external validation.

- **Challenging the Inner Critic:**
  - Self-compassion helps counteract the inner critic, that harsh and judgmental inner voice that can be so critical of oneself.
  - By practising self-kindness and recognising that everyone makes mistakes, you can quiet the inner critic's negative commentary.

- **Cultivating Self-Compassion:**
  - Self-compassion is a skill that can be developed through mindfulness and self-compassion exercises.
  - These exercises may involve self-compassionate self-talk, writing in a self-compassion journal or guided meditation.

- **Self-Compassion and Resilience:**
  - Self-compassion can enhance resilience in the face of

challenges and setbacks.

- It allows you to bounce back from difficult experiences with greater emotional balance and self-acceptance.

- **Self-Compassion in Relationships:**
  - Being self-compassionate can also improve your relationships with others.
  - When you're kinder to yourself, you're often more compassionate and understanding toward others as well.

- **Cultural and Gender Differences:**
  - Cultural and gender factors can influence how self-compassion is practices and expressed.
  - Some cultures may emphasise self-criticism less or more than others and there can be variations in how men and women approach self-compassion.

- **Balancing Self-Improvement and Self-Acceptance:**
  - Self-compassion doesn't mean you become complacent or stop striving for self-improvement.
  - It's about recognising that growth and change can coexist with self-acceptance and self-kindness.

- **Self-Compassion as a Lifelong Practice:**
  - Self-compassion is not a destination but a lifelong practice. It's something that you can continue to cultivate and deepen over time.
  - The more you practice it, the more it becomes a natural response to life's challenges.

Incorporating self-compassion into your life can lead to greater emotional well-being, improved self-esteem and a more positive outlook on yourself and your experiences.

It's a valuable skill that can help you navigate the ups and downs of life with greater resilience and self-acceptance.

10 STRESS REDUCTION AWARENESS

Stress reduction involves various strategies and techniques aimed at managing and reducing the negative effects of stress on your physical and mental well-being.

Stress is a common part of life, but chronic or excessive stress can lead to health problems and decreased quality of life.

Here are some key points about stress reduction:

- **Types of Stress:**
    - Stress can be categorised into two main types: acute stress, which is short-term and often related to a specific event or situation and chronic stress, which is long-term and may result from ongoing challenges, such as work pressure or relationship difficulties.

- **Physical and Mental Effects:**
    - Chronic stress can have a range of physical and mental health effects, including increased risk of heart disease, weakened immune function, anxiety, depression and sleep disturbances.

- **Stress Reduction Techniques:**
    - There are many effective stress reduction techniques

and practices, including:

- **Mindfulness Meditation:**
  - Mindfulness meditation helps you focus on the present moment, reducing anxiety and promoting relaxation.
- **Exercise:**
  - Regular physical activity releases endorphins, which are natural mood lifters.
  - Exercise can also improve sleep and reduce muscle tension caused by stress.
- **Deep Breathing:**
  - Deep, diaphragmatic breathing techniques can activate the body's relaxation response, reducing stress and anxiety.
- **Progressive Muscle Relaxation:**
  - This technique involves systematically tensing and relaxing muscle groups to reduce physical tension.
- **Yoga:**
  - Yoga combines physical postures, breathing exercises and mindfulness to reduce stress and improve flexibility and strength.
- **Tao Chi:**
  - Tao Chi is a mind-body practice that involves slow, flowing movements and deep breathing.
  - It promotes relaxation and balance.
- **Social Support:**
  - Spending time with friends and loved ones, sharing your feelings and seeking support from others can reduce the negative effects of stress.
- **Healthy Lifestyle Choices:**
  - A balanced diet, adequate sleep and limiting the consumption of alcohol, caffeine and nicotine can all contribute to stress reduction.

- **Time Management:**
  - Effective time management techniques can help reduce stress related to work or a busy schedule.

- **Cognitive Behavioural Therapy (CBT):**
  - CBT is a therapeutic approach that helps individuals identify and change negative thought patterns and behaviours contributing to stress and anxiety.
  - It provides coping strategies to manage stress more effectively.

- **Stress Reduction Programs:**
  - Some individuals benefit from structured stress reduction programs or workshops that teach stress management techniques and provide ongoing support.

- **Work-Life Balance:**
  - Achieving a healthy work-life balance is essential for reducing stress. Setting boundaries, prioritising self-care and taking regular breaks can prevent burnout.

- **Mindful Eating:**
  - Practising mindful eating, as discussed earlier, can help reduce stress related to food and improve overall well-being.

- **Nature and Relaxation:**
  - Spending time in natural settings, such as parks or forests, can have a calming effect on the mind and reduce stress.
  - Activities like reading, listening to music or taking a warm bath can also promote relaxation.

- **Seeking Professional Help:**
  - In cases of chronic or severe stress, it's important to

seek help from a mental health professional, such as a therapist or counsellor, who can provide specific strategies and support for managing stress.

- **Regular Practice:**

  - Stress reduction techniques often require regular practice to be effective. Consistency is key to maintaining lower stress levels over time.

It's important to note that what works best for stress reduction can vary from person to person. Experimenting with different techniques and finding what resonates with you is a valuable part of the process.

Reducing stress is not just about avoiding stressful situations but also about developing effective coping mechanisms and resilience to deal with life's challenges in a healthier way.

ABOUT THE AUTHOR

Susan Rogers has been writing resources for the health and social care sector since 2004. Her desire to create balance for hard working staff has resulted in this publication, which is aimed not just at health and social care staff, but everyone.